Praise for
Read again without glasses

"The stuff the optician won't tell you! Leo Angart is an inspirational author and teacher and after 30 years my prescription is being reduced rather than increased. Leo has inspired me to appreciate and exercise my eyes daily and the results are amazing. Just as I've always thought – there really is a natural solution to everything!"

Janey Lee Grace, author of *Imperfectly Natural Woman*

"This book really does offer the opportunity to read again without glasses. At first I thought this was a fanciful idea but the book clearly and eloquently gives evidence to back up the claim. It debunks many of the myths around eyesight which, unfortunately, most people see as true. Having the book and DVD together is great as it offers the next best thing to going to an actual workshop. Even though the exercises are easy to follow they are still very effective. The book and DVD leave you more informed about your specific vision condition, with practical steps as to how to improve it.

"If you are prepared to do the exercises in a non-judgemental way (i.e. by asking how can my eyes improve without laser surgery?) you will definitely reap the benefits.

"I highly recommend this book to anyone."

Anthony Barrett, Co Developer of Sleepora

"Vision training is a vast topic and competence area, mastered by few people. There is powerful scientific material supporting vision training. At the same time our society suffers more than ever from poor vision.

"Leo Angart does important and excellent work throughout the world spreading knowledge of vision training and physiotherapy for the eyes. There is so much every one of us can do in order to see better. This knowledge is indeed precious.

"In this book he shares exactly how you can restore eyesight back to normal, even if you are in your forties and in need of reading glasses. With supportive videos coming with the book, you get all the clarity and inspiration you need. This book itself is a great achievement for mankind and highly recommended."

Ann-Marie Näslund, Founder and CEO of Naturlig Syn, Sweden

Leo Angart

read again without glasses

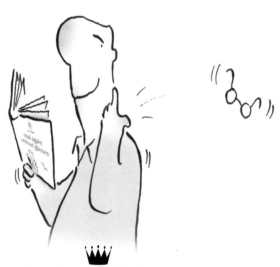

Crown House Publishing Limited
www.crownhouse.co.uk
www.crownhousepublishing.com

First published by

Crown House Publishing Ltd
Crown Buildings, Bancyfelin, Carmarthen,
Wales, SA33 5ND, UK
www.crownhouse.co.uk

and

Crown House Publishing Company LLC
6 Trowbridge Drive, Suite 5, Bethel, CT 06801, USA
www.crownhousepublishing.com

First published 2014.

British Library Cataloguing-in-Publication Data
A catalogue entry for this book is available
from the British Library.

Print ISBN 978-184590891-1
Mobi ISBN 978-184590903-1
ePub ISBN 978-184590904-8
LCCN 2013952191

Printed and bound in the UK by
Gomer Press, Llandysul, Ceredigion

DISCLAIMER
Read again without glasses is not meant for diagnosis and treatment for any medical condition for
the eye or the visual system. The author, publisher and distributor are in no way liable for any
damage whatsoever arising from the use or misuse of this material or the exercises suggested
including but not limited to any personal injury. If you are in any doubt contact your doctor.

Thank you

First and foremost I want to thank William H. Bates, M.D., who in 1912 discovered the possibility of restoring normal reading ability. Dr. Bates is the grandfather of Vision Training as well as the developer of the Bates Method. I also want to thank Arthur Skeffington, one of the founders of Behavioral Optometry, who concluded that the function influences the structure, a basic concept in Vision Training

I would like to recognize the many learning experiences provided by the participants in my workshops around the world. It is a very special feeling when individuals discover that the exercises work and begin to imagine what it would be like to read small print again without glasses.

I also want to thank my collaborators who have made it possible for you to hold this book in your hands: Eva Spitzer, who offered many important suggestions as well as made sure that everything was correct, and Wolfgang Gillesen for always being supportive and making his great experience in this field available. Also a big thank you to Katrina Patterson for organizing more than 40 workshops in London. The pictures and video are the work of the award-winning photographer Lity Sy. A special thank you to Candice Temple for making the book read better by refining my English and to Göchen Eke for his cartoon illustrations that light up the pages. And, finally, thank you to the editors and production staff at Crown House Publishing for publishing this book.

Contents

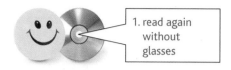

1. read again without glasses

1. Introduction

You have probably picked up this book because you are wearing reading glasses or have been told that you need them.

I wore glasses for 26 years – both glasses for reading and near-sight glasses. This was not because I had presbyopia but because I had -5.5 diopters of near-sight. That is, I could only see clearly to a distance of about 18 cm without glasses. So, I needed one pair of glasses for reading to bring my vision out to a normal reading range of 35 cm and another pair of glasses for distances.

In 1991, I found out how to get rid of my glasses for good. It took me three months to get from the top of the eye-chart to the 20/20 line. My eyesight has been perfect ever since. So I am speaking from personal experience.

Since 1996, I have taught Vision Training classes all over the world. During the last few years, I have developed effective methods for improving even presbyopia that is so severe that *everything* looks blurry without glasses.

This book is my attempt to shine some light on the subject of presbyopia. There are so many misconceptions about it. I have included some of the recent research and, once and for all, exposed some of the myths. The most important myth to debunk is *it's not about age*.

There is a DVD included with this book which includes videos explaining how to perform the exercises. The DVD icon that appears in Chapters 1, 4, 8, 10, 16, 17, 18, 19, 22, 23, 25, 26, 29 and 32 indicates that there is an accompanying video available on the DVD. The disk also includes PDFs of the charts which appear in Chapters 16, 18, 25 and 26. Alternatively, these can be downloaded from the Vision Training website: www.vision-training.com. There is also an interview on the accompanying DVD.

If you are not sure what your vision status is, then it may be better for you to find a time to come to one of my workshops. The advantage is that you will obtain a true picture of the state of your eyesight and, more importantly, what you can do about it. And, of course, you can ask me questions face to face.

I hope that by the time you get through all the exercises in this book, you will once more be able to read without glasses.

2. A Vision Training pioneer

William H. Bates, M.D., the grandfather of Vision Training, was himself severely presbyopic. He cured himself and then went on to develop his own methods of Vision Training. In his book, *The Cure of Imperfect Sight by Treatment without Glasses*, he says:

> The truth about presbyopia is that it is not "a normal result of growing old," being both preventable and curable. It is not caused by hardening of the lens, but by straining to see at the near point. It has no necessary connection with age, since it occurs, in some cases, as early as teen years, while in others it never occurs at all. (1919: 214–215)

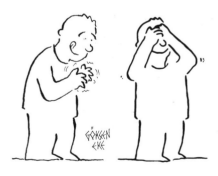

Dr. Bates' main point is that vision problems mainly occur due to mental strain. So, his approach is to relax the eyes by the exercise of "palming." This involves rubbing your hands to warm them, and then using them to cover your closed eyes for a period of time. He also suggested energizing the eyes by allowing the sun to shine on them through closed lids.

3. The road to the discovery of a cure for presbyopia

William H. Bates, M.D., includes an interesting story about how he discovered the cure for presbyopia in an article printed in the magazine, *Better Eyesight*. Dr. Bates writes about an incident that happened around 1912 when a friend asked him to read a letter. To his embarrassment, Bates had to spend some time searching for his reading glasses.

> Being a friend he could say things no other person would say. Among the disagreeable things he said was, and the tone was very empathetic, sarcastic, disagreeable, "You claim to cure people without glasses; why don't you cure yourself?" I shall never forget those words. They stimulated me to do something. I tried all manner of means, by concentration, strain, effort, hard work, to enable myself to become able to read the newspaper at the near point. ...
>
> I consulted specialists in hypnotism, electricity experts, neurologists of all kinds and many others. One I called on, a physician who was an authority in psychoanalysis, was kind enough to listen to my problem. With as few words as

possible I explained to him the simple method by which we diagnose near-sightedness with the retinoscope.

As I looked off into the distance, he examined my eyes, and said that they were normal, but when I made an effort to see at a distance he said that my eyes were focused for the reading distance, i.e. nearsighted. Then when I looked at fine print at the reading distance and tried to read it, he said that my eyes were focused for a distance of twenty feet or farther, and the harder I tried to read, the farther away I pushed my focus. He was convinced of the facts, namely: a strain to see at the distance produced near-sightedness, while a strain to see near produced a far-sighted eye ...

Stumbling on the truth

The man who finally helped me to succeed, or rather the only man who would do anything to encourage me, was an Episcopal minister living in Brooklyn. After my evening office hours I had to travel for about two hours to reach his residence. With the aid of the retinoscope, while I was making all kinds of efforts to focus my eyes at the near point, he would tell me how well I was succeeding. After some weeks or months I had made no progress.

But one night I was looking at a picture on the wall, which had black spots in different parts of it. They were conspicuously black. While observing them my mind imagined they were dark caves and that there were people moving around in them. My friend told me my eyes were now focused at the near point. When I tried to read my eyes were now focused for the distance.

Lying on the table in front of me was a magazine with an illustrated advertisement with black spots which were intensely black. I imagined they were openings of caves with people moving around in them. My friend told me that my eyes were focused for the near point; and when I glanced at some reading matter, I was able to read it. Then I looked at a newspaper and while doing so remembered the perfect black of my imaginary caves and was gratified to find that I was able to read perfectly.

We discussed the matter to find what brought about the benefit. Was it strain, or what was it? I tried again to remember the black caves while looking at the newspaper and my memory failed. I could not read the newspaper at all. He asked, "Do you remember the black caves?" I answered, "No, I don't seem to be able to remember the black caves." Well," he said, "close your eyes and remember the black caves." And when I opened my eyes I was able to read – for a few moments. When I tried to remember the black caves again, I failed.

The harder I tried, the less I succeeded and we were puzzled. We discussed the matter and talked of a number of things, and all of a sudden without an effort on my part I remembered the black caves, and sure enough, it helped me to read. We talked some more. Why did I fail to remember the black caves when I tried so hard? Why did I remember the black caves when I did not try or while I was thinking of other things? Here was a problem. We were both very interested and finally it dawned on me that I could only remember these black caves when I did not strain or make an effort.

I had discovered the truth: *a perfect memory is obtained without effort and in no other way.* Also, *when the memory or imagination is perfect, sight is perfect.* (1922: 1–4; emphasis in original)

Presbyopia is caused by stress, not age. Consequently, if stress and strain are relieved, the ability to read and see at the near point comes back.

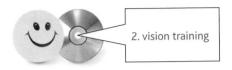

4. Presbyopia – what is it?

If you are reading this book, perhaps with the help of your reading glasses, then you have no doubt heard the common explanation for presbyopia. Either your lens loses its elasticity or the ciliary muscle around the lens loses its power. You are told that this is only to be expected as you get older and, by the way, it's not curable. The only way you will be able to read is with the aid of reading glasses. A depressing scenario.

These theories come from papers written by Helmholtz (1855) and Donders (1864). Helmholtz suggested that presbyopia is caused by a hardening of the lens and Donders thought it was a weakening of the ciliary muscle. These theories are widely believed and often stated as fact.

Some doctors even maintain that they can predict a person's age by measuring the near point of clear vision – the closest you can read clearly. Using this logic, at 45 your near point of clear vision is supposed to be 45 cm and at 50 it diminishes to around 50 cm.

So what are the facts? Several modern studies using modern testing equipment categorically disprove Helmholtz's and Donders' theories.

Hardening of the lens

Firstly, about 63% of the lens is made up of water and there is no noteworthy change with age. Fisher and Pettet (1973) concluded that there is no significant change in the lens with age and that stiffening of the lens is not the cause of presbyopia.

Before cataract surgery, surgeons often use constant ultrasonic speed to accurately predict the required optical power of a lens implant. The speed of ultrasound through the lens is directly related to its elasticity, and the speed of ultrasound through the lens remains constant with age. Schachar et al. (1993) conducted studies on primates with presbyopia. They used ultrasound measurements whilst the animals focused their eyes. They concluded that changes in the lens equator which occur during accommodation involve small displacements of less than 100 microns (100 microns is about the width of one human hair). Schachar (1992) went on to demonstrate that he could reverse presbyopia by sewing a ring around the eye.

Weak muscles

Concerning the strength of the ciliary muscle, Saladin and Stark (1975) studied the power of this muscle and discovered that it actually continues to contract after accommodation is achieved. Tamm et al. (1992) concluded that the power of the muscle would be zero at age 120. In other words, it has power even greater than that required to relax the fibers that hold the lens in place. Fischer (1988) states: "the ciliary muscle undergoes compensatory hypertrophy as accommodation amplitude decreases with age. The force of contraction is about 50% greater at the onset of presbyopia than in youth."

Another factor is that the lens grows in thickness by about 0.02 mm per year, and will be twice as thick at age 80 as it was at age 20. So, the idea that thickening of the lens equates to the loss of the abilities of accommodation or focusing does not really hold up to objective examination. The fact is that we still do not really know the causes of presbyopia.

5. What reading glasses do to your eyes

Most people do not question the widely held assumption that wearing glasses is the best thing that can be done for their eyesight problems. Very few of us take time to consider what really happens when we put glasses on, and why this may not be the best solution.

Vision is not static. Your eyesight is in a constant state of change. This is a fact that most people are familiar with. For instance, all of us have felt our eyes getting tired after a long day in front of the computer.

Glasses are fitted with the purpose of correcting refractive error. In other words, the lens is supposed to focus the image that we see precisely onto the retina. However, glasses compensate for the refractive error in an inflexible way. When worn, the particular level of refractive error must be constantly maintained in order for you to be able to see through them.

This is further aggravated, as is generally the case, if your prescription is for a 100% correction at the exact time of measurement. This is because your eyes will have to adapt to the external conditions at the moment when your eyes were tested. So, if you happen to have your eyes tested in the evening after work, your eyes will always be forced to adapt to those conditions, even if you are walking about in broad daylight. You may have experienced this effect when donning new glasses for the first time, only to find that the prescription hurts your eyes. When you complain about this, the answer is usually, "You will get used to them in a few days."

So how does this continuing saga affect your eyesight? Obviously, your eyes have to keep adapting to maintain the refractive error in exactly the way it was on that evening when your eyes were measured. In other words, your eyesight is forced to deteriorate, just so the glasses will have the correct prescription!

Importance of the optic center

Lenses in all glasses have only one point of best vision – the optic center. This means that because of the way they are constructed, it is as if you are always looking through the dead center of the lenses, with this center located directly in front of your eyes as you look straight ahead. When you look through the glasses and turn your eyes away from this center, the lenses become more like prisms. You have probably seen this effect on photographs taken using wide angle lenses. The edges of the image get distorted. This, along with the fact that glasses also have some sort of frame, encourages you to keep your eyes locked into the position that produces the best vision. A frequently used practice in the attempt to control diverging eyes is the fitting of strong plus lenses. This is a treatment that sadly ends up driving the vision further downhill.

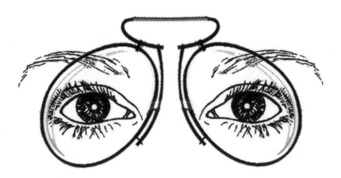

The optic center also plays a role when you use lenses for reading. Remember, your glasses are prescribed with the intention of correcting your distance vision. When you look at the horizon, your eyes point straight out through the optic center of the glasses. However, when you read, you turn your eyes in and down in order for them to converge on your book. Unless you wear special reading glasses, or have them incorporated into your glasses, the optic center of each lens will be further apart than required. The result is additional strain on your eyes – and the more you read the greater the damage.

Does wearing glasses affect the size of your eyes?

Shockingly, there is ample scientific evidence that lenses fitted on young primates do affect the development of their eyes. Whilst conducting research at a New York University, Wallman and Winawer (2004) demonstrated that wearing a minus lens (normally prescribed for near-sightedness) actually causes the elongation of the eyeball; in other words, it causes near-sight to deteriorate. The same is the case with plus lenses fitted for presbyopia or far-sight. This research into emmetropization, the natural ability of the eyes to develop clear vision, goes back to the early 1990s.

Of course, the idea that glasses make your vision worse is resisted by the optical industry. This has ominous overtones, as we all remember how tobacco smoking was not considered harmful by the tobacco companies.

What's annoying about glasses?

Wearing glasses is at best a compromise. Everyone knows that glasses do not provide a solution that gives hassle-free clear vision. They cause many annoying inconveniences. Just remembering where you've put them can drive you to a point of frenzy! And how annoying it is when they fog up as the humidity changes when you go from outside to inside. They also get dirty, scratch or break at the most inopportune moments.

With the Vision Training approach, our objective is to completely eliminate the need for glasses by means of exercises. Our goal is natural clear vision – nothing less.

6. Computer work and reading glasses

Most of us spend a lot of time working at our computers. This means we're looking at a screen for most of the time. The usual distance from eyes to screen is around 60 cm.

Normal reading glasses are designed to be used at an optimum reading distance of 30–40 cm. In other words, reading glasses are not designed to be used for the distance from the screen. It follows that when you use regular reading glasses for computer work you are actually straining your eyes. This will most likely lead to a worsening of your vision and, consequently, the need for even stronger reading glasses. If you must use reading glasses for computer work, they should be fitted for the distance to your screen.

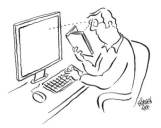

There is another important vision function involved here, the natural resting point, which is the position at which there is no visual input. For example, at night your eyes will find a resting point from where there is no effort in converging or directing your eyes. This resting point is normally about 50–80 cm away from your eyes. If your resting point coincides with the position of your screen, then there is very little effort involved in looking at your screen. However, when the resting point is in front of or behind the screen, you have to constantly use muscle power to force your eyes to converge on the screen. This, of course, leads to fatigue, eyestrain and eventually headaches. For this reason, the best position for the screen is as far away from you as possible. Research shows that you make fewer mistakes when the screen is one meter away than when the screen is closer.

To sum up. Firstly, glasses for computer use should have a lens power that gives you optimum vision at the distance of your computer screen, not for the visual distance you need for reading a book. Secondly, the convergence – the center point of the lenses – should be at the computer screen distance and take into account that your angle of sight is on the screen. In this way, there will be a minimum of stress on your eyes.

Often optometrists do not take enough time to take all these measurements meticulously. If the center of the lens is off by even a millimeter, the plus lenses become prisms that will further strain your eyes while reading. Furthermore, the angle at which you view your screen should also be taken into account. Your near point of clear vision becomes closer as the reading angle moves downwards. If the computer screen is straight ahead of you, your computer lenses should be fitted so that you get optimum vision when looking straight ahead. In other words, the center of the lens should be right in front of your eyes when you are looking at the screen. Off-the-peg glasses are only designed for reading books.

Bi-focal or multi-focal lenses require you to turn your head upward in order to look through the right portion of the lens. Holding this position for long periods of time may lead to neck and shoulder tension or pain.

7. Bi-focal glasses

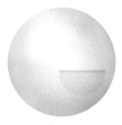

Bi-focal glasses are two lenses fitted together in the same frame. The first bi-focals had a line through the center causing a distinct break between seeing into the distance and reading.

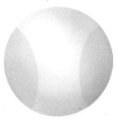

Tri-focal glasses go a step further by incorporating a middle layer through which you view objects in the middle distance. These glasses are also known as vari-focal since there is no distinct line between the differing focal powers of the lens.

Multi-focal glasses incorporate several points of clear vision, which fit into the lens at different angles.

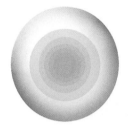 The aim of multi-focal lenses is to provide a smooth transition from distance, to intermediate, to near vision, with in-between corrections as well. You get the best correction when looking directly at the object of focus. There is a corridor of optimum vision that runs vertically down the lens. The optometrist must place the corridor in just the right location in order for you to get optimum vision when you point your nose directly at whatever it is you want to see.

There are many progressive lenses on the market. The differences are mainly in the width of the central corridor of optimum vision. Some lenses are made for computer use and have a wider intermediate zone.

There are also contact lenses with rings of varying focal power. Nowadays you can even get multi-focal lens implants. Always consider having a multi-focal lens implant with great care, since the implant cannot subsequently be removed. At least contact lenses can be thrown away.

Modified mono-vision is an attempt to cover all possibilities by fitting a single power contact lens on one eye and a multi-focal lens on the other. Since not everyone can get accustomed to this, a free trial period is usually included in the offer. However, it can take longer to fit these lenses than normal single power lenses, so there could be extra charges for the fitting.

Bi-focal glasses

Bi-focal or multi-focal lenses are hated by many, especially people who used to have distortion-free vision. Vari-focals sometimes make straight lines look bent, and can cause nausea and dizziness after extended use. In the worst cases, multi-focal lenses can result in a situation where your vision is universally fuzzy: nothing is clear without the glasses. In many instances, your vision has been altered in order to enable you to see through the multi-focal lenses, to a point where you can no longer see anything without glasses, especially if the diopter power is more than +2.5.

A diopter (D) is a measurement of the refractive (light bending) power of a lens needed to correct your eyesight. The strength of prescription glasses and contacts is measured in these units. For reading glasses they are plus (+) lenses or magnifying glasses. For example, a lens that is +0.50 diopters is very weak, whereas a lens that is +4.0 diopters is very strong.

It may require a number of steps in order to gradually restore your normal vision to after wearing multi-focal lenses.

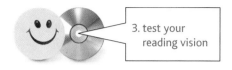

3. test your reading vision

8. Get your eyes tested

It is a good idea to have your eyes tested before you start on your Vision Training program. You will then know precisely what the status of your vision is and how it will register on the eye doctor's equipment. Two tests are normally employed in determining what strength lenses you need to correct your vision to a perfect 20/20. Usually, the optometrist will use a machine to get an objective reading. The machine employs a calculated average, with a plus or minus half diopter margin of error. The machine tests for absolutely perfect focusing at a distance of six meters.

The second test is a subjective test where you look through several types of lenses in order to establish which ones are the most comfortable. This test usually takes place in a room with dim light. Part of the problem with this test is that your eyes keep trying to adapt to the various lenses and, in doing so, you tend to end up with a prescription that is too strong. You have probably experienced coming back the next day and trying on the new glasses, only to find that they hurt your eyes. This is because the glasses have over-corrected your vision and the focus is too sharp for your eyes.

The human eye also varies by as much as 2 diopters in visual acuity during the day. If you measure your vision every few hours, you will find a different reading every time.

9. Visiting the optometrist

Some optometrists are opposed to reducing a prescription to less than the results of their test. If your optometrist belongs to that category, then I suggest you find someone else!

Let the optometrist measure your eyes using his or her instruments. By the way, just measuring your eyes with the automatic equipment is only a rough estimate. The machines vary and have a plus/minus error factor of half a diopter (one line on the eye-chart).

When the optometrist has finished the test, you will have what they determine to be 100% correction of your vision. Usually you will find this to be incredibly sharp and, in some cases, so sharp it actually hurts the eyes. If so, ask the optometrist to reduce the prescription by +0.5 or +1.0 of a diopter. Then go outside into the street and look though the test lenses he has prescribed. It is not enough to just look around in the optometry shop or the shopping mall. You need to see how the glasses work in daylight and while looking at the real world.

For the best results, get a prescription which gives you distance vision that is slightly soft. This will give a correction of about 20/40 distance vision. However, make sure that your prescription is not under-corrected by more than half a diopter. If you reduce the correction more than this, there is a chance that you will actually begin to strain the eyes, in which case your progress in Vision Training will be greatly reduced.

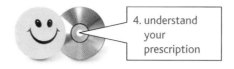

4. understand your prescription

10. Understanding your prescription

The prescription you get from the optometrist looks like Greek to most people. It seems to make no sense whatsoever. Actually it is much simpler than it looks. Firstly, it shows one measurement for the left eye and one for the right eye. Usually this is indicated with an "L" for the left eye and an "R" for the right.

Optique 20/20	Date		Name			Tlf:		
Date:		Sph	Cyl	Axis	Prism	Add	Lens type	
Name:	**Right**	-2.50	0.50	85°				
I.D. No:								
Frame:	**Left**	11.50	-0.50	85°				
Lenses:								
Extras:								
Sub Total:	Contact Lenses	BC	Diam	Power	Solutions		Lens type	
C/L Consult:								
Total:								
Voucher:	Tint	Coating	Type	O.C.	Special instructions			
Deposit:								
Balance to pay:								
	Frame	Model	Size	Colour				

The first column indicates the degree of refractive error (i.e. it tells you whether you are myopic and by what degree). This measurement is indicated in diopters. If you are myopic then there will be a minus indication such as -2.50 D, or minus two-and-a-half diopters. In some countries this is referred to as 250 (they simply drop the period). If you are hyperopic (far-sighted) or presbyopic (need reading glasses) then the indication will be +1.50 D, or plus one-and-a-half diopters. Note that there often is a difference in the prescription for each eye because one eye will be better than the other.

The next column indicates whether there is any astigmatism. When light rays entering the eye do not all meet at the same point (similar to a frayed string) this results in blurred or distorted vision. This is also measured in diopters. The pre-scription will also note in which axis the astigmatism is found. The notation might be something like this: Cyl: -0.5 Axis: 85. This means a cylinder correction of minus one-half of a diopter at an 85 degree axis. Note that it is possible to have astigma-tism in only one eye, or the degree and axis can differ from one eye to the other.

The third column is usually dedicated to divergence. The read-ing for strabismus (when one eye turns in or out) is usually corrected using "prism elements." These are indicated in prism diopters and the letter D is often used to indicate that a prism element is included.

There will generally be a space on the form for any additional notes from the optometrist. Sometimes near vision will also be tested, and there may be a prescription for bi-focal lenses.

Another possibility is that you will be given a prescription for glasses with variable focus lenses that have two or three areas with different lens power. Suggested lenses and frames are also often noted.

The slips of paper that are printed out from machines used to check visual acuity also show other numbers that are relevant if you are being fitted with contact lenses.

Once you have had your eyes tested you are ready to go ahead and start your Vision Training. You will probably notice an improvement quite quickly. This is your subjective experience of vision, which is always ahead of the objective measure. You might be able to actually see and read four or five more lines on the eye-chart, but the machine will not show any improvement at all. The machine measures only absolutely perfect focusing, not the fact that you can see better than before.

Do yourself a favor and carry on with your Vision Training exercises for about a month before you go for another eye test. However, during that period you may need to have the power of your lenses reduced, since the old prescription will no longer be relevant and the lenses may start to hurt your eyes.

11. Can exercises help you to see?

Your eye care professional will most likely say no, it's just not possible for exercises to improve your vision. Since optometry is mainly about selling glasses, this response is understandable. To their chagrin, optometrists are already losing business, with reading glasses now going for a song in stores and supermarkets.

The prevailing belief is that accommodation (or focusing) of the eye cannot be learned. Yet everyone knows that you can practice your golf swing or your tennis serve and expect your game to improve. In other words, training leads to superior performance. This is a concept we are all familiar with. So why shouldn't it be the case with our eyes? After all, accommodation or focusing also involves muscles.

The eyes have an accommodative range. This is the range within which we can see clearly. This range is dynamic and constantly changing. You have probably had an experience of this after a long day at work – noticing that your vision is worse in the evening than it was in the morning, when you felt less tired.

There is no denying that things change as we get older. Our energy and stamina tend to lessen. We need more rest and move at a slower pace. As far as the eyes are concerned, we begin to feel the limits of our accommodative (visual) range around our mid-forties.

Fortunately, our accommodative range can be trained. The reason this is possible is that our focusing system, just like other parts of our bodies, operates by means of muscle power. As everyone knows, muscle power and flexibility can be improved and trained. This book teaches you exactly how to do this for the sake of your eyesight.

If life was balanced so that you used near vision and distance vision more or less equally, you would be likely to maintain good eyesight for most of your life. People who work in the countryside, on farms or the like, often have good eyesight. For instance, in native societies in South America and other areas where life centers around hunting, people's eyesight is often exceptionally acute.

When we say we have 20/20 vision, this refers to the ability to see 827 mm high letters on an eye-chart 6 meters away. This is a measurement of how well you see at a distance – also known as visual acuity. It is sometimes converted to decimal by dividing the numbers, so perfect vision becomes 1.0. It can also be expressed in metric notation so that perfect vision will be 6/6 or 100%. All the notation systems express the same measurement.

Normal visual acuity with age
after Elliot et al., 1995

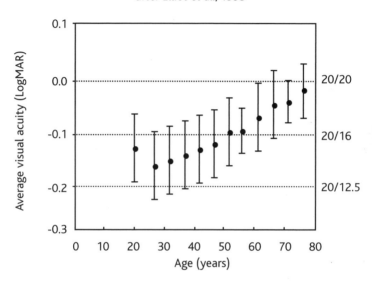

Most existing studies concern eyesight problems. However, there is a study which tracks the progress of "normal" eyesight through a lifetime. Elliott et al. (1995) found that normal eyesight at age 24 is about 20/14. Vision naturally slowly deteriorates as we get older, so at age 75 normal vision is 20/19.

12. Relax and see

Natural clear vision is effortless – you simply open your eyes and see. Problems arise when we begin to force our visual system. As we grow up, and especially when we start going to school, we learn to repress our natural internal signals. For instance, if a 4-year-old child feels sleepy, she will start to rub her eyes. This is a signal that she needs rest. Somewhere along the way she will learn to repress this natural urge, especially when she gets a bit older and starts wearing make-up! Tension starts to build up in the visual system as we begin to use more force to accomplish visual tasks. Or we simply continue reading way past the time when the eyes need a break.

Near-point tension develops when we attempt to hold the focusing system steady – for instance, on the book in which we are engrossed – for too long. Research shows that even short periods of stress require several hours of recovery. This may explain the relationship between academic achievement and vision. Sadly, a doctorate is often accompanied by the onset of myopia, also known as short-sightedness or the inability to see at a distance.

13. Vision Training and presbyopia

The idea behind Vision Training is very simple. As mentioned above, everyone knows that training improves performance. So, the focus of Vision Training is to restore the normal function of the eyes by means of a series of specific exercises.

The first problem with presbyopia is that the near point of clear vision slowly creeps further and further away. Little time will have elapsed before your arms just aren't long enough! We want to bring this near point backwards so you can once again read clearly at about 15 cm from your eyes.

The second problem is that reading small print becomes more and more difficult. Usually this is the reason you go and buy reading glasses in the first place. So, you need to train your eyes to read small print again. There is an exceptionally effective Vision Training exercise that can do just that.

The third problem is that, as time marches on, you tend to require more and more light in order to be able to read. This is connected with the decrease in visual power as well as with the opening up of the iris. The less light there is available, the more the iris opens up, so that sufficient light will fall on your retina for you to be able to see the text. The larger the opening, the more blur will be apparent if your eyes do not have much focal power (amplitude of accommodation) left.

When we train the eyes, we start off by reading small print in daylight, as this is obviously easier. We then train the eyes to read in progressively lower and lower light. And train them for different kinds of light conditions. If you can read 3-point type in candlelight, then you will have no problem reading in any other surroundings.

14. What kind of presbyopia do I have?

Your ability to read is tested by reading a "reduced" eye-chart. You have perfect near vision if you can read 4-point print from a distance of 35 cm. The numbers in the left-hand column of the near-vision eye-chart indicate the font size used in the passages of text.

Note that the quality of light has a great influence on your reading ability. Indoors, in the evening, your visual acuity will drift up a line or two. Ideally, you should be able to see the 20/20 or 4-point line clearly at about 15–20 cm in front of your eyes. This is normal visual acuity for activities at the near point. Children can see print at about 5 cm from their eyes.

Near-vision test

If you have 20/20 vision for reading then you should be able to read the lines below in good daylight at a normal reading distance (about 35 cm):

20/50 (9pt) A b C d E f G h I j K 1 3 5 7 9 2 4 6 8

20/40 (8pt) A b C d E f G h I j K 1 3 5 7 9 2 4 6 8

20/30 (6pt) A b C d E f G h I j K 1 3 5 7 9 2 4 6 8

Your reading vision may be OK for most situations; however, you may have difficulty in low-light situations.

20/25 (5pt) A b C d E f G h I j K 1 3 5 7 9 2 4 6 8

Your reading vision is pretty good – just a fraction below the optimum.

20/20 (4pt) A b C d E f G h I j K 1 3 5 7 9 2 4 6 8

Congratulations, you have perfect near-point reading vision.

The basic idea is that you need to have extra energy or stamina, so that when your eyes get tired you will still be able to read at a comfortable reading distance.

The significance of the near point

Normally the near point should be about 15 cm from the eyes. If your near point is further out than that, it shows that you are probably presbyopic. In any case, you need to do exercises that will bring your near point back to, or very close to, 15 cm. Presbyopia occurs when you have difficulty reading but still have excellent distance vision. If your near point of clear vision is more than 25 cm out, then you should start doing the presbyopia exercises in the reading small print exercise (see Chapter 16). 5 \

15. Measure your amplitude of accommodation

This measurement estimates your visual power. A normally sighted 10-year-old child has about 20 diopters of visual power and can see clearly about 5 cm in front of his or her nose. Visual power slowly declines with age, mostly due to damaging visual habits. We tend to work most of the time with a focal distance limited to the computer screen or to the machine we are working with. Doing this for years causes the visual system to adapt to the environment in which we find ourselves. Also, the relationship between energy and muscle power slowly diminishes as we grow older.

When you were 18 years old, you could go out dancing all night and not be fazed by an all-night party the next day after school or work. If you try this today you will definitely notice the lack of sleep! Around the age of 45 we begin to notice a lack of flexibility in our visual system. Our visual power will have fallen to about 5 diopters, and you have to hold the newspaper at arm's length to read it. If you only attempt to correct this by donning reading glasses, sadly you will not be doing anything to improve matters – you are passively accepting your fate and your vision will most likely continue to deteriorate.

To measure your own amplitude of accommodation, take this book and bring it as close as you can to your eyes whilst still being able to read perfectly. Measure the distance in centimeters from your eyes to the book.

Divide this figure by 100 and you will have your "amplitude of accommodation." For example, if the closest point at which you can read this book without glasses is 50 cm, then your amplitude of accommodation is: 100/50 = 2.0 diopters.

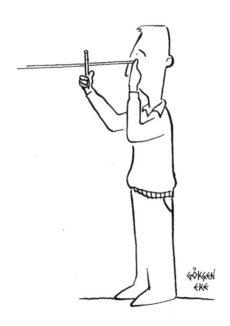

The idea is to improve your amplitude of accommodation; that is, to bring your near point of clear vision in closer. Generally you will want to achieve a near point of clear vision as close as possible to 15 cm in front of your eyes. In Chapter 16 there is a small print exercise which you can use to determine your near-vision acuity.

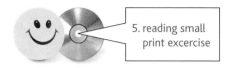

5. reading small print excercise

16. Reading small print exercise

Note: A printable chart in the correct size is included on the DVD. Alternatively, you can download the reading exercise from www.crownhouse.co.uk/featured/Read_Again or use the text on the following pages.

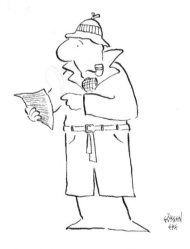

This exercise should be done with good daylight illuminating the page. First read as far down the page as you can. Then turn the page upside down and start to scan the white space between the lines. As you do so, imagine that the background is a brilliant white, like sunlight reflected on water or snow. Keep your breathing nice and deep. Continue to scan the white spaces as if you were reading. Go all the way to the bottom of the page. Now, turn the book the right way up and see how many more words or paragraphs you can read.

There is no need to read each paragraph – it's the same text in different font sizes. Continue this exercise for five minutes or until you can read to the bottom paragraph; that is, read it from any distance within arm's length. You will first notice that words appear to become clear, and then sentences and finally the whole paragraph. For some people this process is very rapid but others will need to practice quite a few times before can they relax enough to allow their eyes to adjust. It is about allowing yourself to explore the possibility of developing more flexibility and discovering how it would look and feel. It's an intriguing question, isn't it – how would I feel if I could read print this small?

Persons whose sight is beginning to fail at the near point, or who are approaching the so-called presbyopic age, should imitate the example of a remarkable old gentleman I met. Find a sample of really small print and read it a few times every day. Start in good daylight then use different kinds of artificial light, bringing it closer and closer to the eyes until it can be read at a distance of about 15 cm or less. Or get your own sample of type reproduced to several incrementally smaller sizes, and use the same technique. By practicing this exercise, you can not only escape the necessity of wearing reading glasses, but hopefully also avoid many of the eye troubles that so often afflict people. Nature intended you to have natural clear eyesight.

Persons whose sight is beginning to fail at the near point, or who are approaching the so-called presbyopic age, should imitate the example of a remarkable old gentleman I met. Find a sample of really small print and read it a few times every day. Start in good daylight then use different kinds of artificial light, bringing it closer and closer to the eyes until it can be read at a distance of about 15 cm or less. Or get your own sample of type reproduced to several incrementally smaller sizes, and use the same technique. By practicing this exercise, you can not only escape the necessity of wearing reading glasses, but hopefully also avoid many of the eye troubles that so often afflict people. Nature intended you to have natural clear eyesight.

Persons whose sight is beginning to fail at the near point, or who are approaching the so-called presbyopic age, should imitate the example of a remarkable old gentleman I met. Find a sample of really small print and read it a few times every day. Start in good daylight then use different kinds of artificial light, bringing it closer and closer to the eyes until it can be read at a distance of about 15 cm or less. Or get your own sample of type reproduced to several incrementally smaller sizes, and use the same technique. By practicing this exercise, you can not only escape the necessity of wearing reading glasses, but hopefully also avoid many of the eye troubles that so often afflict people. Nature intended you to have natural clear eyesight.

Persons whose sight is beginning to fail at the near point, or who are approaching the so-called presbyopic age, should imitate the example of a remarkable old gentleman I met. Find a sample of really small print and read it a few times every day. Start in good daylight then use different kinds of artificial light, bringing it closer and closer to the eyes until it can be read at a distance of about 15 cm or less. Or get your own sample of type reproduced to several incrementally smaller sizes, and use the same technique. By practicing this exercise, you can not only escape the necessity of wearing reading glasses, but hopefully also avoid many of the eye troubles that so often afflict people. Nature intended you to have natural clear eyesight.

Persons whose sight is beginning to fail at the near point, or who are approaching the so-called presbyopic age, should imitate the example of a remarkable old gentleman I met. Find a sample of really small print and read it a few times every day. Start in good daylight then use different kinds of artificial light, bringing it closer and closer to the eyes until it can be read at a distance of about 15 cm or less. Or get your own sample of type reproduced to several incrementally smaller sizes, and use the same technique. By practicing this exercise, you can not only escape the necessity of wearing reading glasses, but hopefully also avoid many of the eye troubles that so often afflict people. Nature intended you to have natural clear eyesight.

Persons whose sight is beginning to fail at the near point, or who are approaching the so-called presbyopic age, should imitate the example of a remarkable old gentleman I met. Find a sample of really small print and read it a few times every day. Start in good daylight then use different kinds of artificial light, bringing it closer and closer to the eyes until it can be read at a distance of about 15 cm or less. Or get your own sample of type reproduced to several incrementally smaller sizes, and use the same technique. By practicing this exercise, you can not only escape the necessity of wearing reading glasses, but hopefully also avoid many of the eye troubles that so often afflict people. Nature intended you to have natural clear eyesight.

Persons whose sight is beginning to fail at the near point, or who are approaching the so-called presbyopic age, should imitate the example of a remarkable old gentleman I met. Find a sample of really small print and read it a few times every day. Start in good daylight then use different kinds of artificial light, bringing it closer and closer to the eyes until it can be read at a distance of about 15 cm or less. Or get your own sample of type reproduced to several incrementally smaller sizes, and use the same technique. By practicing this exercise, you can not only escape the necessity of wearing reading glasses, but hopefully also avoid many of the eye troubles that so often afflict people. Nature intended you to have natural clear eyesight.

Persons whose sight is beginning to fail at the near point, or who are approaching the so-called presbyopic age, should imitate the example of a remarkable old gentleman I met. Find a sample of really small print and read it a few times every day. Start in good daylight then use different kinds of artificial light, bringing it closer and closer to the eyes until it can be read at a distance of about 15 cm or less. Or get your own sample of type reproduced to several incrementally smaller sizes, and use the same technique. By practicing this exercise, you can not only escape the necessity of wearing reading glasses, but hopefully also avoid many of the eye troubles that so often afflict people. Nature intended you to have natural clear eyesight.

Congratulations, if you can read this comfortably in both artificial light and in daylight then you have 20/20 near vision. To maintain your near vision you need to read small print like this or smaller at least a few times every month. Take something you are really interested in reading and use a photocopy machine and have the magazine or article reduced to small print like this. Then read it with regular light and with just one candle. You can have a glass of wine as a reward. When you are reading with the absolute minimum light possible, you are training your visual system to function comfortably with very low light. Now go and find the darkest spot in the room and read this again. How did it go? Do this about once a week from now on and you eyesight will be fine for the rest of your life.

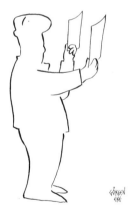

The next step is to check what difference there is, if any, between your eyes. Look at one of the small print paragraphs that you can read comfortably. Close your left eye. If you need to move the book to read comfortably, then you will know that there is a difference between your eyes. Now, switch eyes and look at the small print with your right eye. Again, if you need to move the book there is a difference.

To equalize the reading distance between your eyes, close the eye that can read the closest. Move the book to the point where the other eye can read the text clearly. To encourage the eye to adjust, begin to move the book just a little bit closer, so that the text starts to become blurred. The eye will now attempt to adjust for the slight difference and, in most cases, succeed in doing so. Continue this backwards and forwards movement until your eyes can read at the same level.

Finally, you will want to train your eyes to read in a variety of light conditions. In bright daylight the cone cells are active and will provide you with crystal clear vision. In low light you will need to use more of the rod cells which are highly sensitive to light. You naturally move from one type of cell to another and have the ability to read small print in very low light conditions.

When you can read the paragraph above printed in the smallest font size in good daylight, then progress to reading it in lower and lower light levels. Move from outside to inside and notice how this changes your ability to read. Continue to practice at different light levels until you can read fine print with just one candle.

Reading small print upside down is the most important exercise to do in order to get rid of your reading glasses. Do this exercise as often as you can (aim for 50 times a day for just 30 seconds). Go from small print to large print just once. The aim is to get more flexibility into your visual system. How do you get more flexible? You exercise, of course.

Often this exercise is the clincher for people. It is proof that they can succeed. Finding that you can, all of a sudden, read tiny print also motivates you to continue your practice and make the improvements permanent.

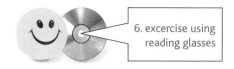

6. excercise using
reading glasses

17. Using reading glasses
as a tool

Often people in my workshop tell me that *nothing* is clear. They can't see even the largest letters without glasses. This is usually the case if the reading glasses get to +2.5 diopters or more. It is also often the outcome of wearing multi-focal glasses or contact lenses. The eyes adapt to the glasses, so that when you remove them you can't see anything.

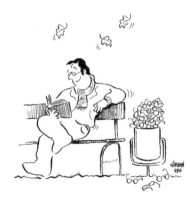

Not being able to see anything clearly is obviously quite distressing. However, there is hope for people whose sight has deteriorated to a point where they cannot read anything without glasses. Simply start using those inexpensive off-the-peg reading glasses you can buy from supermarkets, drug stores or chemists. Buy a pair of glasses where you can read 12-point print clearly – this will be your starting point.

Both the near-vision and small-print exercises can be done just as effectively with reading glasses.

Do the reading small print exercise with your new reading glasses until you can read 4-point print. When you can read 4-point print then your glasses are too strong for you. Go and buy another pair with lower diopters. Find a pair where you can just read 12-point clearly. Do the read small print exercise with your new lower power reading glasses until you can read 4-point print again.

Gradually work your way through glasses with lower and lower strength until you can read 4-point print with +1.0 diopter glasses. Then you can begin to read the larger print clearly without glasses. Continue doing the exercise until you can read the smallest print in daylight.

If there is a difference between your eyes, then do the exercise with only the weaker eye. Repeat the exercise until you can read the same line with both eyes.

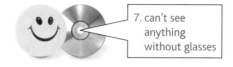

18. If you can't see anything without glasses

When the power of your reading glasses exceeds +3.5 diopters your vision may begin to change until you can't see anything without the glasses. Multi-focal glasses can have the same effect. A participant in my workshop in Vienna, Austria said she found it beyond frustrating.

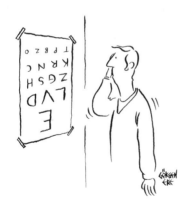

Sometimes it is only one of your eyes that can't read small print. If this is the case, then you need to do the exercise with that particular eye only. Print off an eye-chart (one can be downloaded from www.crownhouse.co.uk/featured/Read_Again or can be found on the accompanying DVD) and work through the list below. Make sure you find the smallest letters you can read perfectly, but do not compromise – the text must be

can read perfectly, but do not compromise – the text must be absolutely clear. You want your brain to know that you want clear vision, not just less blur.

1. Find the smallest letters you can see perfectly clearly with your right eye.

2. Do the same with your left eye. If there is a difference between your two eyes then do the exercise with the eye that can read the largest letters until you can read the smallest print with both eyes.

3. Turn the eye-chart upside down.

4. Scan the lines of white space between the letters. Do this all the way down to the bottom of the page.

5. Turn the page the right way up. You will notice that the letters get darker and eventually become clear.

6. Continue this until both eyes can read the same line with the same clarity.

7. Next, continue the exercise until you can read the bottom line of the eye-chart.

If your presbyopia has advanced to the point where your reading glasses are +3 or +4 diopters then you won't be able to read anything without glasses. If this is the case, then you will need to start with baby steps and begin by simply using old reading glasses with lower lens power.

Choose a pair of reading glasses with which you are able to read midway down the eye-chart. Do the exercise with the old reading glasses until you can read the bottom line with those glasses.

The most important step is to make both eyes capable of reading the same line. Once you can do this, the next step can be done with supermarket reading glasses, which always have the same prescription for both eyes.

Continue doing this exercise, with reading glasses of lower and lower diopters, until you can read the bottom line of the eye-chart without any glasses.

If you need glasses for driving, then get yourself a pair of glasses that have been prescribed specifically for driving. Discard your bi-focal or multi-focal glasses. This will make things a bit more complicated since you will have to buy another pair of glasses. However, most people do not drive for long periods of time, so it is just a small compromise.

When you have accomplished reading the bottom line of the eye-chart without reading glasses, you are ready to start on the reading small print exercise (see Chapter 16).

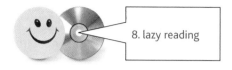

19. Lazy reading exercise

The purpose of this exercise is to develop flexibility in focusing between the near point and far point, as well as sharpening your focusing powers. This exercise also develops the ability to read smoothly without regressing.

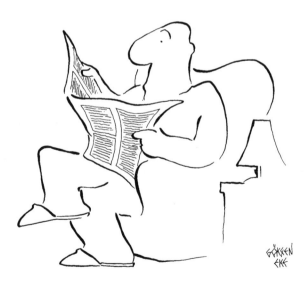

1. Find a book or a magazine which has plenty of white space between the lines and a typeface that appears slightly blurred when you hold the page out in front of you.

2. Turn the page upside down so that you cannot read the text.

3. Run your eyes gently and slowly around the margins a few times, looking as if from the back of your head.

4. Now choose two points at the top corners of the page, and another point, such as a box of tissues, at a distance within the room.

5. Shift your eyes from the page to the box then back and forth.

6. Next, scan the white spaces between the lines, scanning down the page as if you were reading. By the time you are halfway down, everything may seem clearer, but do not strive for clarity – keep on going.

7. When you reach the bottom, turn the book or magazine right side up, and look along the white space below the first line of type.

8. Close your eyes now, and from memory paint imaginary white in the space below the first line of type, then look back and forth between the text and the white space.

9. Open your eyes and scan the spaces beneath the first few lines, imagining them as being bright as snow in brilliant

sunlight. Repeat this several times, alternately closing and opening your eyes.

10. Now, float your eyes back and forth over the lines without reading.

11. Look away, then return to the page. The black of the type will seem blacker, and the white of the spaces will seem whiter than you have ever seen them. The words will stand out sharply.

Devote 15 minutes a day to this exercise. In the weeks that follow, gradually reduce the size of type you practice with until you are able to easily read small print.

The lazy reading exercise involves many activities and is therefore a great stimulus for both mind and visual system. Like the small print reading exercise (see Chapter 16), lazy reading also relies on the foreground/background principle. For example, if you look at wallpaper with a flower pattern you can pick one flower and bring that into the foreground, whilst the overall design remains in the background.

When we read, we naturally see the black text in the foreground, since this is what we are focusing on. Switching the two around frees up the mind to do other work and we experience a relaxation of the visual system. This gives us the ability to see the text much more clearly.

20. When there is a large difference between each eye

To eliminate the difference between each eye, you need to work on the eye that has the worst vision; that is, the one that requires reading matter to be held at the greatest distance.

A disparity in reading distance between your eyes often leads to eyestrain and headaches. It is therefore important to eliminate any differences there may be in the reading distance of each eye. One gentleman in Sydney, Australia was so thankful that he had discovered the reason he always became tired while reading. After practicing to balance his reading vision, the tiredness and headaches disappeared, even when reading for long periods.

21. How to check your near point for reading

1. Take any piece of text that you can read without glasses (e.g. the eye-chart).

2. Slowly move the text as close as you can to your eyes, whilst still maintaining absolutely clear vision in both eyes.

3. Close your left eye. If you need to move the page outwards to keep it clear then there is a difference.

4. Repeat the process with your right eye closed and find out how closely you can read with perfect clarity.

5. You may discover that one eye is very different from the other in ability. If this is the case, then you need to use large print, such as an eye-chart, to train that eye to read smaller and smaller print.

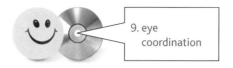

22. Eye coordination and reading

The ability of our eyes to work together develops within the first few months of life. This is the vergence, or triangulation, of your two eyes as they point towards the object you are looking at. The vergence usually remains unchanged as the near point moves away from you. However, sometimes your point of convergence will slowly drift out of alignment. This is a very gradual process which you are usually not aware of. If your point of convergence is either in front of or behind the object you are looking at, your eyes will become stressed. You may see a slight doubling which can give an impression of fuzziness and hence become confused with near-sight. At the most extreme, your brain may even temporarily switch one of your eyes off.

Eye coordination works best when both eyes have the same visual acuity. If there is even a small difference, your visual system will become stressed. In some laser surgery operations, doctors will give one eye good reading vision and the other the right prescription for driving and seeing into the distance. This is known as mono-vision but some people cannot get used to it.

How to test for convergence

Convergence is one of the easiest things to check and correct. Take a piece of string, about the length from hand to hand when stretched across your chest (about 1.25 meters). Tie the string to the back of a chair or to a door handle. Next you will need a paperclip or a bead, which you can slide up and down the string.

1. Place the loose end of the string at the tip of your nose so that the string is stretched out.

2. Place the paper clip somewhere in the middle of the string.

3. When you look at the paperclip you should see two phantom lines crossing directly through the paperclip. If you see the cross in front of the paperclip then your eyes are under-converging. If you see the cross beyond the paperclip then your eyes are over-converging – they are pointing too far. If you see only one string, this means that one eye is suppressing the image. The brain is only heeding one image and is blocking the affected eye – in effect, you are only using one eye. Such misalignment contributes to your vision problem and makes images blurry.

In some cases, the outer eye muscles are too tight and refuse to allow the eyes to move inwards. If this is the case, practice looking at your finger whilst you move it in from arm's length till it physically touches the tip of your nose. When looking at something up close, your eyes move in towards the nose.

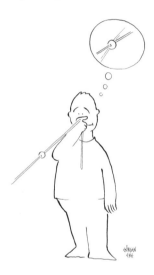

How to improve convergence

Aligning your convergence point is easy. Simply move the paperclip in or out until it coincides with the cross point of the "X." In some cases people see a "V, "A" or "Y" – any of these are fine, as long as the convergence point is directly through the paperclip. When the paperclip is located at your fusion point, begin to move it back and forth while holding the fusion point through the paperclip. If you move the clip slowly, your brain will begin to align your eyes so that they point directly to what you want to see. This is a recalibration and your brain will begin to automatically fuse your vision perfectly.

All the mind needs is a reference and it will automatically make the adjustments for you. Do this exercise for a few minutes only, but do it several times a day, about ten times, until you can easily place the center of the cross anywhere on the string. Look away and look back, still keeping the cross through the paperclip. At this point you will have perfected the exercise and achieved perfect convergence. In my experience, which tallies with research findings, this adjustment takes place quite rapidly and is highly effective. Research suggests more than 85% efficacy.

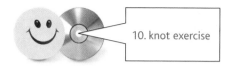

23. Knot exercise

This exercise is designed for developing perfect convergence. Take a string and measure off 2 meters. Next, tie knots every 10 cm along the string. To make the knots stand out you can paint them with colored markers. Alternatively, you can tie on colorful beads or small plastic rings. Colored paperclips would also do.

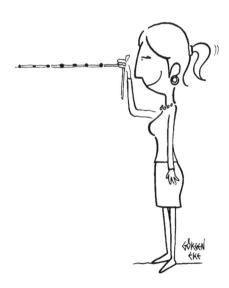

To perform the exercise, tie one end of the string to a door handle or to the back of a chair. Take the free end of the string and put it on the tip of your nose. Keep the string straight and look down its length. You will see a cross centered over every knot you look at. Move your attention from knot to knot and notice how the cross keeps jumping. Vary the exercise, looking at every second knot, every third knot and so on. Also, look away and find the cross again instantly. Develop the ability to see the cross when you look up, down and to the side. Do this exercise about five times a day until you can do it effortlessly – then you will have perfect convergence.

24. Convergence and reading

I often come across people with presbyopia where convergence is a big part of the problem. For one reason or another, the eyes develop difficulty in turning inward. Often the outer eye muscle is held too tight. Perhaps it is because their parents told them not to cross their eyes when they were children. In fact, to read properly, your eyes need to turn inwards (converge) a few degrees. If not, your near point of clear vision will drift further and further away and you will develop presbyopia.

Convergence can be corrected optically using prisms. A prism bends the light towards its base and thereby corrects the divergence. The disadvantage of using prisms is that they quickly become very heavy. Also, there are limitations to the range of vision divergence that a prism can compensate for. Prisms are mostly used for treating strabismus and, of course, the prism will do nothing for the underlying convergence problem.

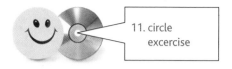

11. circle
excercise

25. Circle exercise

Note: A printable chart is included on the DVD. Alternatively, you can download a chart from www.crownhouse.co.uk/featured/Read_Again or it can be found on the accompanying DVD.

This exercise will teach your centering muscles to work in partnership with your focusing muscles. Usually, when the muscles you use to cross your eyes lack tone, you will automatically over-focus and your near point will be pushed out beyond the page you are reading. This can lead to presbyopia and astigmatism.

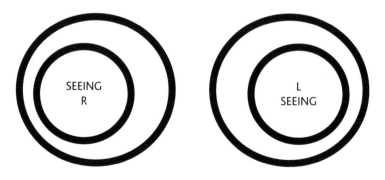

Position this page so that the circles are very close to your eyes. The left and right circles will float together and form a 3D image in the center. The inner circle now floats above the outer circle like a multilayered cake. The word SEEING floats on top and you will see two words one above the other.

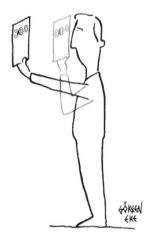

If you see the "R" and the "L" that means your fusion is not quite complete. The perfect alignment shows the word SEEING in two lines, perfectly aligned one above the other. No "R" and no "L" is seen. Keep this image and slowly move the book away from you until it is at arm's length. You should be able to maintain the convergence and the image in perfect focus at all distances from about 15 cm to arm's length. Next, look away and back again. You should be able to regain the fused image instantly. Practice for a few minutes at a time, and frequently, until you can easily see the image. If your eye muscles become sore then stop the exercise. This is about developing flexibility, so be gentle.

Next, hold the diagram at your normal reading distance and begin to slowly move the page in clockwise circles, progressively making larger and larger circles. Do the same counterclockwise. This will train your ability to keep convergence across the printed page.

Eventually you should be able to get perfect convergence from close up to arm's length. You should also be able to look away at something in the distance, then switch back and see the perfectly fused image instantaneously. Once you can do this you can stop doing the circle exercises.

This is what you should see.

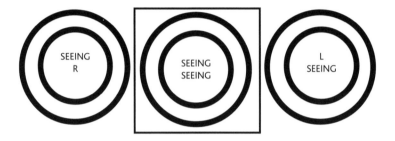

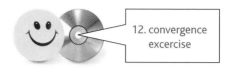

12. convergence excercise

26. Combining convergence and visual acuity

Ray Gottleib, O.D., Ph.D. – one of the pioneers of Vision Training – combined a convergence exercise with a visual acuity test. Gottleib did this in the late 1970s and has thereby helped countless people to maintain their ability to read. It is further evidence that presbyopia is not inevitable.

Here is a similar exercise that will help you to maintain your reading vision. There are two ways to do this exercise.

Exercise 1: with two dots

Note: A printable chart (convergence excercise 1) is included on the DVD. Alternatively, you can download a chart from www.crownhouse.co.uk/featured/Read_Again

1. Hold the chart out at arm's length.

2. Place a finger halfway between yourself and the chart. Look at the tip of your finger.

3. In the background you will see a column of text recessed behind the other two columns. The image will be in 3D (similar to the magic pictures that were popular in the 1970s).

4. Relax, take a deep breath and begin to read the text. You will notice that it becomes clear as your brain adjusts to the eyes' convergence. This exercise can be very strenuous, so practice it for brief periods only, until your visual system starts to strengthen. Approach it as play, rather than exercise.

Sight is mind and eye coordination.

It is more mental than physical. The eye sees but the mind must interpret and evaluate what is seen.

There are five basic components of mental sight: curiosity, contrast, comparison, memory and judgment.

Curiosity means intelligent visual searching, that is, looking around just as if you saw everything with perfect clarity.

Counting objects and colours is the best way to achieve curiosity.

Contrast is the gradations of difference between foreground and background.

not to scale

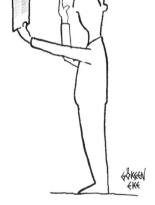

5. When the image becomes clear at arm's length, slowly remove your finger and begin to gradually move the chart back and forth until you can read it at as close a distance as possible. Make a note of which numbered block of text you can now comfortably read.

This is what you should see.

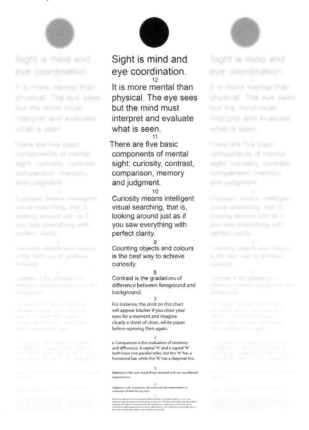

Sight is mind and eye coordination.

12
It is more mental than physical. The eye sees but the mind must interpret and evaluate what is seen.

11
There are five basic components of mental sight: curiosity, contrast, comparison, memory and judgment.

10
Curiosity means intelligent visual searching, that is, looking around just as if you saw everything with perfect clarity.

9
Counting objects and colours is the best way to achieve curiosity.

8
Contrast is the gradations of difference between foreground and background.

7
For instance, the print on this chart will appear blacker if you close your eyes for a moment and imagine clearly a sheet of clean, white paper before opening then again.

6
6 Comparison is the evaluation of similarity and difference. A capital 'H' and a capital 'N' both have two parallel sides; but the 'H' has a horizontal bar, while the 'N' has a diagonal line.

5
Memory is the sum total of our learned and our recollected experiences.

4
Judgment is the summation, the end result, the interpretation or evaluation of what the eye sees.

Exercise 2: with four dots

Note: A printable chart (convergence exercise 2) is included on the DVD. Alternatively, you can download a chart from www. crownhouse.co.uk/featured/Read_Again

1. Hold the chart very close to you and look between the four dots.

2. Relax, and you will see a fifth column, in 3D, floating out towards you.

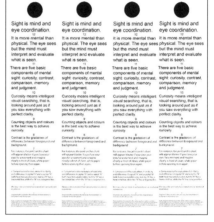

3. Begin to move the chart back and forth, gradually moving it out to arm's length. If you lose the effect, go back to where you can see the 3D column and begin, little by little, moving the chart back and forth, working slowly, until you get to arm's length.

4. Read as far down as possible. Make a note of which numbered block of text you can now comfortably read.

This exercise can also be quite strenuous, so go slowly. Do it for brief periods only, until your visual system has build up convergent strength.

This is what you should see.

Sight is mind and
eye coordination.
12
It is more mental than
physical. The eye sees
but the mind must
interpret and evaluate
what is seen.
11
There are five basic
components of mental
sight: curiosity, contrast,
comparison, memory
and judgment.
10
Curiosity means intelligent
visual searching, that is,
looking around just as if
you saw everything with
perfect clarity.
9
Counting objects and colours
is the best way to achieve
curiosity.
8
Contrast is the gradations of
difference between foreground and
background.
7
For instance, the print on this chart
will appear blacker if you close your
eyes for a moment and imagine
clearly a sheet of clean, white paper
before opening them again.
6
o Comparison is the evaluation of similarity
and difference. A capital "H" and a capital "N"
both have two parallel sides but the "H" has a
horizontal bar, while the "N" has a diagonal line.
5
Memory is the recollection of our likeness and our recollective
experiences.
4
Judgment is the common interpretation of our recollective
evaluation of all that we see.

27. What is the best light for reading?

Of course, daylight is the best of all because it contains the entire spectrum of colors, but it is not always possible to read in daylight. So, the question is really: what is the optimum source of artificial light? For industrial purposes, daylight can be reproduced artificially by a variety of methods. They include wide-band fluorescent, 7 phosphor wide-band fluorescent and filtered tungsten/halogen light. At a cost, all these lighting technologies can reproduce light with a color spectrum very similar to daylight. The energy content of a light source determines our ability to see colors accurately. So it is important to choose light that reproduces daylight as closely as possible.

Daylight is measured by three standards: D55 represents daylight at noon, D65 is average daylight and D75 is the standard northern sky. All three standards have a similar spectral content.

28. What is color temperature?

Color temperature is a measurement that indicates the hue of a specific light source. British physicist William Kelvin conducted an experiment whereby he heated up a block of carbon. As it glowed in the heat, it produced a range of different colors as the temperature increased. First it produced a dim red light, increasing to a brighter yellow as the temperature went up. Eventually it became a bright blue-white glow at the highest temperatures. In his honor, color temperatures are measured in degrees of kelvin (K).

Lower color temperatures contain more red and appear warmer, whereas higher color temperatures contain more blue and appear cooler. The flame of a lighted match is 1,700–1,800 K. Candle light has a color temperature of 1,850–1,930 K. Standard light bulbs have a fairly yellow light with color temperatures around 2,700 K. Daylight bulbs have a much bluer light around 6,000–6,500 K. Direct sunlight has a color temperature of 5,000–5,400 K. Daylight, on a partly cloudy day, is much bluer and has a color temperature of 8,000–10,000 K.

Color temperature is best known for its application in color films. To get natural looking colors indoors, you need to choose whether to take pictures with outdoor film using 5,500 K or indoor film with 3,200 K color temperature. Using a 3,200 K indoor film to take pictures outside will result in images that are too blue. Using a 5,500 K outdoor film indoors will result in images that are too yellow. Color temperature also changes with the weather. Pictures taken on an overcast or rainy day need a warm filter to make them look natural.

Color Rendering Index

The Color Rendering Index (CRI) is a measurement of how accurate colors appear under a specific light source. The CRI is measured on a scale of 1–100. Light with just one color has a rating of 1, whereas natural sunlight has a CRI of 100. For example, standard daylight tubes have only moderate color rendering with a CRI of around 75. To get closer to real daylight, special light-emitting diode (LED) lights are available, which can be dimmed as well as alter color temperature from yellow (2,500 K) up to blue (6,500 K). It is possible to get LED light sources exceptionally close to natural sunlight with a CRI of 96 or even 99.

What is color temperature?

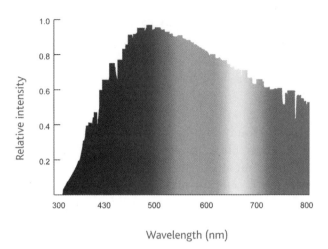

Wavelength (nm)

N55 color spectrum of daylight with CRI of 99

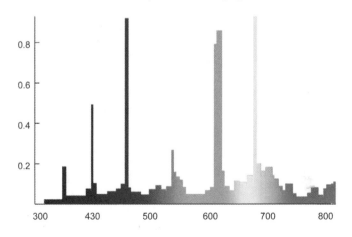

Color spectrum of typical fluorescent light with CRI of 70

How do we perceive white?

Color temperature and the intensity of the ambient light determine how we perceive colors. On a sunny day, the light level measures 13,600 foot candles (the light from one candle, placed one foot away) and 5,000 K. In this light we perceive pure white. If it is a cloudy day, the light measures about 3,200 foot candles and has a color temperature of 6,650 K. When we move indoors, or at night, the iris opens wider and more of the light sensitive rod cells are at work. Since rod cells have a higher sensitivity to blue, we perceive the light source as bluish, while 4,700 K appears white.

If you go into a museum, the light level is usually further reduced by a factor of 10 from about 200 to 20 foot candles. The rod cells are used even more and 4,700 K now appears bluish or cold while 3,500 K appears white.

It is important to note that as the iris changes in size, the actual image on the retina does not change. Thus, for a given field of view, such as reading, the same numbers of rod and cone cells are exposed. It is the amount of light which triggers a larger visual influence of the cone cells for higher illumination and the rods for lower illumination.

The overall environment also affects the perception of color. For example, if you introduce a small beam of daylight into a room illuminated by incandescent light, it will appear bluish, because your eyes will be adjusted to the lower light level which activates more blue orientated rod cells.

What is the perfect artificial light source?

The best artificial light sources are LEDs because they can be manufactured to have a color spectrum that comes the closest to the D55 standard. For the best results, you need to choose the color temperature that is most suitable for your light level.

For indoor use, like an office, look for a bulb of 4,700 K. If you want a lower light level for computer work, then consider a 4,100 K or 3,500 K bulb. The basic idea is to make white appear white in all light conditions and thus the most comfortable for your eyes.

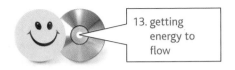

29. Chinese acupressure
for the eyes

There are ten steps to this exercise. Its purpose is to get the energy flowing through your eyes and head. You may notice that some of the pressure points feel slightly tender. This indicates that energy is not flowing very freely at that particular energy point. The massage movement will start things moving again and you will feel a wonderful freshness and openness after this exercise.

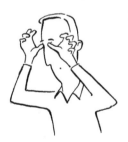

1. The first point – bladder meridian B2, which improves eye problems – is located at the root of the nose and up under the eyebrow. Place the tip of your thumb as close as possible to the inner corner of the eye and press upwards. You will sense a tender spot right where the point is located. Rotate gently three times either right or left. Alternatively, just press and release several times.

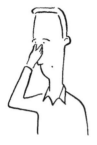

2. The second point – bladder meridian B1, which also improves eye problems – is located on each side of the root of the nose, right where the petals of your glasses normally rest. Use your thumb and index finger and grip the root of your nose. Make gentle circular movements. Alternatively, you can just press and release.

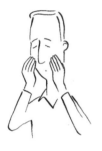

3. The third point – stomach meridian ST 3, which improves cataracts and swelling under the eyes – is located on the cheekbone at the same level as your nostrils, about one-and-one-half fingers outwards. Use three fingers and you are sure to touch this point. Do gentle circular movements. Alternatively, you can also just press and release.

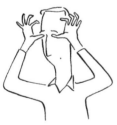

4. The fourth step involves several acupuncture points along the bone over your eyes (gallbladder GB 2 and triple warmer). Begin where you found the first point, then move outwards in small steps across the bone to the outer corner of the eye.

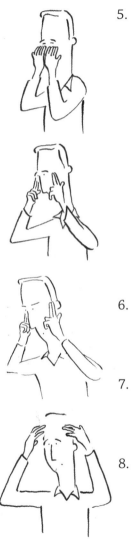

5. Next comes the bone under the eye. At the inner corner of the eye we have the first point of what is known as the bladder meridian. Directly underneath the center of the eyeball we have the first point of the stomach meridian, ST 1, which relieves red eye, night-blindness, over-active tear ducts and also near-sight. The easiest way to do this is to use four fingers and press down and release on the edge of the bone. Sometimes you will feel a wonderful coolness flowing down over your eyes indicating the flow of energy.

6. The next step is the gallbladder GL 1 point located at the outer corners of the eye. Massage with gentle circular movements.

7. Next, move to the hairline and the TW 22 point on the triple warmer. Massage with gentle circular movements.

8. Move a bit further back, placing your fingertips on an imaginary vertical line moving up from the ears. Massage the four points

beneath your fingertips. This is the gallbladder meridian. Massage with three circular movements right to left (counterclockwise). Then energize with left-to-right clockwise movements.

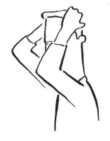

9. This movement is often referred to as the "tiger climbing the mountain." Open and close your fingers as if they were claws – the movement you use when you are washing your hair. Start from the hairline and move up and back towards the center of the head, using one long, smooth movement. You can use the soft part of your fingers (if you have long finger nails) or you can use your nails. Put some pressure on to get the energy flowing. With this one movement you stimulate more than 15 acupuncture points on each side of your head.

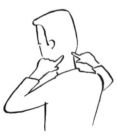

10. The final point is located at the back of the head, just where your neck muscles are attached to the skull. You will find some indentations on each side of your head – this is where the 20 gallbladder points are

located. Massage with gentle
circular movements.

This energy moving exercise can be used as many times as you like. It is especially useful when you feel that your head is getting a bit woolly because it gets the energy moving around your eyes and head. It also stimulates a plethora of beneficial acupuncture points. I also suspect that it may encourage hair growth. It is an exercise that you can practice for almost any vision problem and experience positive results.

30. Relieving tired eyes

People who have the symptoms of presbyopia often tend to strain their eyes. Fortunately there is a simple way to draw tension out of the eye muscles. You will need two small towels of a size similar to the ones you get in Chinese restaurants before or after dinner.

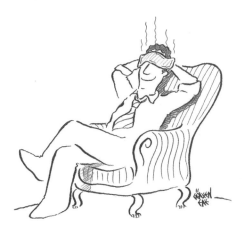

1. Dip one towel in hot water – as hot as you can stand it. Wring the water out and place it on your closed eyelids for about ten seconds.

2. Take another towel and dip it in cold water. It does not have to be icy cold – just cold tap water. Place this on your closed eyelids for a few seconds.

3. Repeat this three times. The heat will penetrate into your eyes and soften the muscles. The cold will revive the blood circulation and help transport away any blood waste or lactic acid that has built up in the muscles.

The hot-and-cold towel treatment not only feels very good but it refreshes your eyes. Do this once a day for a few days until your eyes start feeling better.

31. What about dry eye?

Dry eye syndrome is associated with long hours at work in dry air from central heating or air-conditioning units. The eyes can feel dry and gritty or even as if there is a foreign body in the eye. The syndrome is actually a collection of symptoms that stem from an imbalance in the quality and quantity of tears.

The balance of tear production and tear loss, through evaporation and drainage, maintains the moisture level in the eyes. Tears are produced by two different methods. One produces tears at a slow, steady rate and is responsible for normal eye lubrication. The other produces tears in large quantities in response to irritation or emotions.

Anatomy of the tear film

Each time you blink, tears bathe and lubricate the eyes. The tears are produced by glands above each eye. The tear film consists of a delicate balance of three layers: an oily layer, a watery layer and a mucus layer.

The *oily layer*, produced by the meibomian glands, forms the outermost surface of the tear film. Its main purpose is to smooth the tear surface and reduce evaporation. Some paints contain a slow-drying solvent, so that the paint dries from the bottom up. The meibomian glands work in a similar way, stopping bubbles forming on the tear surface.

The *watery middle layer* is 98% water and is produced by the lachrymal glands. It cleanses the cornea and washes away foreign particles or irritants.

The *mucus layer* is produced by the conjunctiva. Mucus allows the watery layer to spread evenly over the surface of the eye and helps the eye to remain moist. Without the mucus, tears would not adhere to the eye. It acts as a bonding layer.

What causes dry eye?

Tear production normally decreases with age. Although dry eyes can occur in both men and women at any age, women are most often affected. This is especially true after the menopause. One of the most common causes is extensive use of computers. Computer users forget to blink their eyes and as a result develop dry eyes. Other causes are contact lens wear and, more recently, laser surgery.

A wide variety of common medications, prescription and over-the-counter drugs, can cause dry eyes by reducing tear production. This is especially so in the case of:

- Diuretic drugs commonly used to treat high blood pressure
- Antihistamines and decongestants
- Beta blockers
- Sleeping pills
- Birth control pills
- Tricyclic antidepressants
- Isotretinoin-type drugs for the treatment of acne
- Opiate-based pain relievers such as morphine

Laser treatment can also considerably aggravate dry eyes. People with dry eyes are often more prone to the toxic side effects of eye medications, including artificial tears. For example, the preservatives in certain eye drops and artificial tear preparations can irritate the eye, thus creating a need for special preservative-free artificial tears.

How is dry eye measured and treated?

Several tests can be carried out to determine if you have dry eyes. For example, the Schirmer test involves placing filter-paper strips under the lower eyelids to measure the rate of tear production under various conditions. Another test uses a diagnostic drop (fluorescein or rose bengal) to detect staining patterns in the eyes. This gives the optometrist an idea of where the dry patches are located in each eye.

The most common treatment is artificial tears, which are available over the counter. If you need to use such eye drops more than every two hours, then preservative-free preparations are the best choice.

A natural alternative

There are two basic types of essential fatty acids (EFAs): omega-3 and omega-6. An ideal diet should include a ration of four parts omega-6 to one part omega-3.

Omega-6 fatty acids are found in raw nuts and seeds (and their oils), borage oil, primrose oil, soybean oil, whole grains and legumes.

Omega-3 fatty acids are found in cold water fish, such as salmon, mackerel, sardines and herring. They are also found in walnuts, flaxseeds and canola oil. A deficiency in vitamin A often shows up in the eyes – firstly as night blindness and secondly as a dryness of the conjunctiva (the white part of the eye). Vitamin A is found in carrots, broccoli leaves, kale, sweet potatoes and all forms of liver.

Here is the recommended regimen for improving dry eyes using additional oil intake: take 10,000 international units (IUs) of vitamin A per day (the safe daily limit) to make sure your conjunctiva stays nice and moist. The easiest way of getting the required amount of omega oils is to take four tablespoons of walnut oil or flaxseed oil – both contain the two kinds of omega oils in the right ratio. In addition, take three capsules of evening primrose oil (500 mg) a day.

Note that the oils should be taken cold. If heated they produce harmful free radicals. Walnuts produce a very light oil that is delicious on salads. Eating enough good oils will not only improve your dry eye condition, but also make your skin much softer.

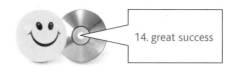

14. great success

32. In conclusion

I hope you will find the time to do the exercises in this book and restore your ability to read again without glasses. I have been presenting Vision Training workshops around the world for more than 18 years, during which time I have seen people significantly reduce their lens power and often get rid of their reading glasses entirely. The exercises presented here are those that I have found to be the most effective.

The common perception is that reading glasses are inevitable as a result of getting older. This is based on Helmholtz's 19th century theory that the lens inside the eye does all the focusing. Modern research using up-to-date equipment and methods has come to different conclusions. However, most eye-care professionals still say that presbyopia can only be corrected with glasses. If we think of Vision Training as physiotherapy for the eyes, it suddenly becomes obvious that you can train the focusing abilities of the eyes. Focusing, like any other physical ability, will respond to the appropriate exercises.

I wish you great success with your exercises and hope that you will enjoy reading again without glasses.

Glossary

20/20 Vision This refers to the ability to see 8.27 mm high letters on an eye-chart 6 meters away. This measurement of visual acuity is sometimes converted to decimal by dividing the numbers, so perfect vision becomes 1.0. It can also be expressed in metric notation so perfect vision will be 6/6. All the notation systems express the same measurement.

Accommodation (focusing) The eye's ability to adjust its focus. When this accommodation skill is working properly, the eye can focus and refocus quickly and effortlessly, which is similar to a very fast automatic focus feature on a camera.

Amplitude of accommodation (AA) A measurement of the eye's ability to focus clearly on objects at near distances. The focusing range for a child is usually about 5–7 cm (2–3 inches). For a young adult, it is 10–12 cm (4–6 inches). The focus range for a 45-year-old adult is considered to be about 50 cm (20 inches.) For an 80-year-old adult, it is 150 cm (60 inches.) However, with Vision Training you can maintain your near-point focus.

Astigmatism Light rays entering the eye do not all meet at the same point (similar to a frayed string), which results in blurred or distorted vision. An abnormally shaped cornea typically causes this condition. Occasionally astigmatism exists in the lens of the eye.

Auto-refractor A sophisticated measuring device that usually includes a keratometer (for measuring astigmatism) as well as a tool to estimate refractive errors. However, auto-refractors do not measure accurately enough to prescribe glasses. An auto-refractor test is often the first procedure performed by an optometrist.

Axis This is the third column on your prescription and indicates the angle where the optometrist will make correction for astigmatism.

Behavioural optometrist (also called a functional optometrist or developmental optometrist) An optometrist who specializes in all aspects of vision as it is related to an individual's development and to the role of vision in relation to reading, computer monitor use and sports. Behavioural optometry has its origins in orthoptics, which is a non-surgical treatment for strabismus. Behavioural optometry's emphasis is on prevention, re-mediation, re-habilitation and enhancement.

Better Eyesight A newsletter published by William Bates from July 1919 to June 1930. Bates and others wrote about his Vision Training work.

Bi-focal glasses These are used to correct vision at two distances and are composed of two ophthalmic lenses, such as a plus lens for near vision and a minus lens for distance vision.

Chinese acupressure A version of acupuncture using the fingers, rather than needles, to apply pressure to acupuncture points.

Ciliary muscle A band of muscle and fibers that is attached to the lens which controls the shape of the lens and allows it to accommodate (change focus).

Color Rendering Index A scale from 1–100 illustrating how natural colors look under a particular light source. The closer you are to 100 the better. Ordinary fluorescent light usually has a CRI of 83 and halogen light has a CRI of 100.

Color temperature The kelvin (K) scale was named after British physicist William Kelvin and is a measurement of the hue of a light source, which is related to the temperature of the light-producing element. Lower color temperatures are more red/orange whilst higher color temperatures are more blue. For example, the flame of a lighted match is about 1,700 K whilst sunlight has a color temperature of 5,000 K. Our perception of color is influenced by the intensity of the ambient light. The eyes compensate automatically so colors look the same in all light levels.

Computer screen distance Your computer screen is usually about 60 cm away from you. Reading glasses are normally designed for about 40 cm. In other words, the optimum vision of reading glasses is about 20 cm too short. If you work like this for any length of time your eyesight is likely to suffer.

Cone cells Light sensitive cells located in the retina. There are three types of cone cells which enable color vision: these are red-, green- and blue-sensitive. The cone cells are concentrated in a 1.5 mm area at the macula where you have perfectly clear vision.

Convergence The ability to use both eyes as a team and to be able to turn the eyes inward to maintain single vision up close.

Cylinder lens An ophthalmic lens that has at least one non-spherical surface and which is used to correct astigmatism. The values are typically from -0.75 to -1.25. The cylinder measurement is given with a minus (-) sign. (Please note that the sign for myopia (near-sightedness) is also a minus.)

Daylight Light emitted by the sun. There are three standards describing true daylight: D55 is daylight at noon in mid-summer, D65 is northern light and D75 is average light. Daylight can be reproduced artificially, usually for industrial applications like color printing, paint making, cosmetics, etc. Light bulbs labeled daylight may not emit a true daylight spectrum of colors.

Diopter (D) A measurement of the refractive (light bending) power of a lens or a prism (pd). The strength of prescription glasses and contacts are measured in these units. For example, a lens that is +0.50 D is very weak, whereas a lens that is +4.0 D is very strong.

Divergence The ability to use both eyes as a team and be able to turn the eyes out toward a far object.

Dry eyes A condition caused by lack of oil in the tear film. There is an outer oil layer floating on the surface of the tear film covering your eyes. When there is a deficiency in the oil, the tears dry up in spots which can make the eyes feel gritty.

Dynamic vision Our eyesight constantly changes as we shift from one distance to another and from side to side as we look around.

Emmetropization A process that controls the growth of children's eyeballs. The diameter of the eye of a baby is about 17 mm. Over the first 15 years, the eye gradually grows to an adult size of 24 mm. Research shows if lenses (plus or minus) are placed in front of the eyes then the lens becomes part of what controls the growth of the eye. A minus lens will make the eye grow longer, thus making the near-sightedness worse. Plus lenses have the opposite effect.

Equalized reading distance If there is a difference in the near point for reading this may cause eyestrain, leading to fatigue and eventually headache. Ideally, both eyes should read at the same distance. Some doctors suggest that you can use one eye for reading (near vision) and the other for distance viewing. However, not everyone can get used to this. With this compromise you may also lose some of your ability to judge distance accurately.

Eye-chart The Dutch ophthalmologist Hermann Snellen designed a chart consisting of letters of various sizes. The normal vision letter height is 827 mm when viewed from a distance of 6 meters. Each line on the eye-chart represents a 5% difference. The second line is considered as 100% visual acuity when viewed from 6 meters. Note: The eye-chart must be at least 5 meters away during visual acuity testing. If not, you will not get an accurate measurement and your glasses may be over-prescribed.

Far point This is the furthest you can see absolutely clearly. The far point measured in centimeters is used to calculate which diopter lens power is needed to correct your eyesight.

Fluorescent light A common light fixture based on vaporized mercury which has a very spiky output of light in just a few frequencies. This makes the light deficient in some of the colors of the spectrum. To remedy this, manufacturers use a variety of phosphorous coatings. Fluorescent lights can flicker unless high frequency fixtures are used.

Foot candles A foot candle is a measurement of the light intensity of one candle when one foot away. The light output of a lamp is often stated in foot candles (i.e. how many candles would be needed to produce the same amount of light).

Fusion The union of images from each eye into a single image. There are three degrees of fusion: 1st degree fusion is the superimposition of two dissimilar targets, 2nd degree fusion is flat fusion with a two-dimensional target and 3rd degree fusion is depth perception (stereopsis) with a three-dimensional target.

Incandescent light The light produced by a traditional light bulb containing a heated tungsten wire. This type of bulb produces a yellow/orange light.

Kelvin Named after British physicist William Kelvin. It is a measurement of the color temperature of a light source. In an experiment, Kelvin heated pure carbon and noticed that it glowed with different colors as it was heated. Kelvin's observation became the norm for describing the color temperature of a light source.

LED light This is the next evolution of light using light emitting diodes which are more energy efficient than other technologies. LEDs are available in red, blue and green, so pure white light can be produced. LEDs are currently available as flash lights but will soon replace all energy saving lights. They use as little as 10% energy compared to ordinary bulbs.

Lens (also referred to as the crystalline lens) A transparent disc located behind the iris which changes shape to focus on objects at different distances from the eye.

Lens implants These are normally used after extracting a cataract. Implants are available with a single power as well as a multi-focal power design.

Lumen The measurement of the perceived power of a light. This is a measurement that is often used together with lux to describe the level of illumination in a given area (e.g. lumen per square foot or lumen per square meter). There are about 10.764 lumens to 1 lux.

Minus (-) lens A concave lens which stimulates focusing and diverges light. The lens is thinner in the center than the edges. It is used in glasses or contact lenses for people who are near-sighted (myopic).

Multi-focal When two or more lenses are integrated into one unit. The simplest form is bi-focal where there is an upper lens for distance viewing and a lower lens for reading. Lenses are also manufactured with three or more focal points. They are often referred to as vari-focal.

Near point This is the closest you can see perfectly clearly. The near point in centimeters is used to calculate your amplitude of accommodation or your visual focusing power. The nearer you can read the better.

Near-vision test chart For near-vision tests a reduced Snellen eye-chart is used. You should be able to read 5 point print.

Objective refraction This is the part of your visual exam that is measurable with equipment such as an auto-refractor or a retinoscopy. The other part of your visual exam is subjective, meaning it is based on your feedback.

Omega 3/Omega 6 Essential fatty acids needed by the body, especially if you have dry eyes. Omega 3 and 6 are found in nut, seed and fish oils.

Optic center The absolute center of a lens must be positioned directly in front the eye. If misaligned the lens becomes more and more prism-like which can cause the coordination of your eyes to be affected. In order to overcome this, your eyes have to use more energy which may eventually lead to eyestrain and headaches.

Optometrist A health care professional who is licensed to provide primary eye care services. These services include comprehensive eye health and vision examinations; diagnosis and treatment of eye disease and vision disorders; the detection of general health problems; the prescribing of glasses, contact lenses, low vision rehabilitation, vision therapy and medications; the performing of certain surgical procedures; and the counseling of patients regarding their surgical alternatives and vision needs as related to their occupation, vocation and lifestyle. An optometrist has completed pre-professional undergraduate education in a college or university and has had four years of professional education at a college of optometry, leading to a doctor of optometry (O.D.) degree. Some optometrists also complete a residency.

Palming William Bates' unique palming exercise is used to relax the visual system. Rub your hands together for a few seconds, then cover your closed eyes – without touching – for about one minute. You will notice that your vision has improved. You are experiencing the Bates relaxation effect.

Plus (+) lens Convex lenses (thicker in the middle) relax focusing and converge light. They are typically used in glasses or contact lenses for people who need reading glasses or are far-sighted (hyperopic).

Prescription Your optometrist will give you a written prescription showing the result of your vision test. The prescription is used to manufacture glasses or contact lenses. It will include measurements for the sphere indicator, cylinder, axis and prism.

Prism A wedge-shaped lens which is thicker on one edge than the other. This plastic or glass lens bends light (in the opposite direction to the thicker end). A prism is sometimes added to glasses to help improve eyesight due to an eye misalignment or visual field loss.

Progressive lenses A lens is progressive when two or three lens powers are seamlessly worked into one lens. These lenses have different designs for different purposes. Mostly they are aimed at computer users with a wider area for the middle range where the computer screen is located.

Reading distance The normal reading distance is considered to be 35–45 cm from your eyes. Reading glasses are normally designed for that distance. *13¾ – 17¾*

Reading vision Our eyes are at rest when we look at the horizon. When we turn our eyes in and down to read, we also alter our natural distance vision by -3 diopters so we can see the book. This is one of the main reasons why near work, such as reading and computer work, may lead to vision problems.

Refraction The optometrist will do an objective refraction or test of your visual acuity. This is done with an auto-refractor or with a retinoscope. The subjective refraction test is done with a refractor, a device containing many lens elements that can be switched in and out. In order to determine your prescription both test needs to be done.

Resting point When you look into the night there is no visual stimulus. Your eyes will revert to a natural "resting point" where there is no muscular effort. This is the optimum resting point – normally about 50–80 cm away. Far-sighted people have a resting point further away, at 150–180 cm.

Retinoscopy This technique determines the eye's refractive error and the best corrective lenses to be prescribed. An instrument called a retinoscope, which consists of a light, lens, mirror and handle, is used to shine light into a patient's eye. When light is shone into the eye, the light is reflected back ("reflex"). If the reflection is in the same direction ("with movement") as the retinoscope then the refractive error is hyperopia (far-sightedness) and a plus lens is prescribed. If the reflection is in the opposite direction ("against movement") to the retino-scope then the refractive error is myopia (near-sightedness) and a minus lens is prescribed. The strength of the prescription is determined when the pupil is suddenly filled with light ("neutralized") by the appropriate lens power (strength).

Rod cells Light-sensitive cells located in the retina. Rod cells are very light sensitive and are used mainly for low light and night vision. These cells are also more sensitive to blue light which is what makes glare (high blue-content light) uncomfortable.

Sphere This is the first line on your prescription and indicates the power of the lens needed to correct your vision. A minus sphere is used for near sight and a plus sphere is used for reading glasses or far sight.

Subjective refraction This is usually the last step in your eye test where the optometrist will try different lens power configurations and ask you which one is clearest. It is based on your feedback since only you can see if the chart is clear.

Tear film The uppermost layer of your tears consists of an oily layer. If you do not have sufficient oils in your diet then you may experience dry eyes. The other two layers are a watery layer and a mucus layer.

Tired eyes Most of us have experienced tired eyes at one time or another. Sleeping is often not enough to relax tired eyes.

Tri-focal When there are three lens elements incorporated into one unit. Typically there is an upper area with good distance focus, a middle band where indoor or the middle ground is in focus (such as when shopping) and a third element which is designed for reading or near work.

Vergence To turn the eyes horizontally (convergence – inward, or divergence – outward). Accommodative vergence, fusional vergence, proximal vergence and tonic vergence are needed to maintain the appearance of a single image.

Vision Training The fact that eyesight is controlled by muscles means that visual ability and function is trainable. Vision Training is a collection of exercises designed restore your vision to normal.

Zonule fibers Tiny fibers in which the lens is suspended like a tent. These fibers pull the lens and make it thinner or more elongated when the ciliary muscle is contracted.

Bibliography

Adler-Grinberg, D. (1987). Questioning our classical understanding of accommodation and presbyopia. In I. Stark and G. Obrecht (eds.), *Presbyopia*. New York: Professional Press, pp. 250–257.

Alpern, M., Mason, G. L. and Jardinico, R. E. (1961). Vergence and accommodation. V: Pupil size changes associated with changes in accommodative vergence. *Am J Ophthalmol* 522: 762–767.

Angart, L. (2005, 2012) *Improve Your Eyesight Naturally*. Carmarthen: Crown House Publishing.

Atchison, D. A., Claydon, C. A. and Irwin, S. E. (1994). Amplitude of accommodation for different head positions and different directions of eye gaze. *Optom Vis Sci* 71: 339–345.

Bates, W. H. (1919). *The Cure of Imperfect Sight by Treatment without Glasses*. New York: Central Fixation Publishing.

Bates, W. H. (1922). Presbyopia. *Better Eyesight* VI(2): 1–4.

Beers, A. P. A. and van der Hoide, G. L. (1994). In vivo determination of the biomechanical properties of the component elements of the accommodation mechanism. *Vision Res* 34: 2897–2905.

Ciuffreda, K. J., Kellndorfer, J. and Rumpf, D. (1987). Contrast and accommodation. In L. Stark and G. Obrecht (eds.), *Presbyopia*. New York: Professional Press, pp. 116–122.

Donders, F. C. (1994 [1864]). *On the Abnormalities of Accommodation and Refraction of the Eye*, tr. U. V. D. Moore. London: New Sydenham Society.

Duane, A. (1925). Are the current theories of accommodation correct? *Am J Ophthalmol* 8: 196–202.

Elliott, D. B., Yang, K. C. H. and Whitaker, D. (1995). Visual acuity changes throughout adulthood in normal, healthy eyes: seeing beyond 6/6. *Optometry & Vision Science* 72: 186–191.

Fincham, E. F. (1955). The proportion of the ciliary muscle force required for accommodation. *J Physiol* 128: 99–112.

Fisher, R. F. (1969). The significance of the shape of the lens and capsular energy changes in accommodation. *J Physiol* 201: 21–47.

Fisher, R. F. (1971). The elastic constants of the human lens. *J Physiol* 212: 147–180.

Fisher, R. F. (1973). Presbyopia and the changes with age in the human crystalline lens. *J Physiol* 228: 765–779.

Fisher, R. F. (1977). The force of contraction of the ciliary muscle during accommodation. *J Physiol* 270: 51–74.

Fisher R. F. (1988). The mechanics of accommodation in relation to presbyopia. *Eye* 2: 646–649.

Fisher, R. F. and Pettet, B. E. (1973). Presbyopia and the water content of the human crystalline lens. *J Physiol* 234: 443–447.

Fisher, R. F. and Pettet, B. E. (1988). Mechanics of accommodation in relation to presbyopia. *Eye* 2: 646–649.

Gottlieb, G. L., Corcos, D. M., Jarie, S. and Agarwal, G. C. (1988). Practice improves even the simplest movements. *Exp Brain Res* 73: 436–440.

Helmholtz, H. (1855), Über de akkommodation des Auges. *Albrecht von Graefes Arch Opththalmol* 1: 1–89.

Helmholtz, H. (1966 [1866]) *Treatise on Physiological Optics*, tr. J. P. C. Southall. New York: Dover.

Hirsch, M. J. and Wick, R. E. (eds.) (1960). *Vision of the Aging Patient: An Optometric Symposium*. Philadelphia, PA: Chilton Co.

Saladin, J. J. and Stark, L. (1975). Presbyopia: new evidence from impedance cyclography supporting the Hess-Gullstrand theory. *Vision Res* 1(5): 537–541.

Schachar, R. A. (1992). Cause and treatment of presbyopia with a method for increasing the amplitude of accommodation. *Ann Ophthalmol* 24(12): 445–447.

Schachar, R. A., Hunag, T. and Huang, X. (1993). Mathematic proof of Schachar's hypothesis of accommodation. *Ann Ophthalmol* 25(1): 5–9.

Storey, J. K. and Rabie, E. P. (1985). Ultrasonic measurement of transverse lens diameter during accommodation. *Ophthalmic Physiol Opt* 5: 145–148.

Tamm, S., Tamm, E. and Rohen, R. W. (1992). Age-related changes of the human ciliary muscle: a quantitative morphometric study. *Mechanisms of Ageing and Development* 62(2): 209–221.

Wallman, J. and Winawer, J. (2004). Homeostasis of eye growth and the question of myopia. *Neuron* 43(4): 447–468.

About the author

Leo Angart is Danish but has lived most of his life in Asia. He describes himself as an "International Dane." Since 1996 he has conducted Vision Training workshops all over the world,

Leo is also interested in the scientific understanding of how the eyes work and especially how you can train the function of the eyes. He is the author of *Improve Your Eyesight Naturally* (2005, 2012).

With this book, Leo has looked into presbyopia – what presbyopia is and the science related to it – and, especially, exercises that are effective for reversing the effects of presbyopia. This includes what you can do if you can't read anything without glasses because your eyes have adapted to powerful reading glasses.

Leo Angart is interested in helping you to regain your natural eyesight. For more information about workshops near you, please visit www.vision-training.com.

Disc menu

Film files

PDF files